I0471154

Future Research Needs Paper

Number 25

Intravascular Diagnostic Procedures and Imaging Techniques Versus Angiography Alone in Coronary Stenting: Future Research Needs

Identification of Future Research Needs From Comparative Effectiveness Review No. 104

Prepared for:
Agency for Healthcare Research and Quality
U.S. Department of Health and Human Services
540 Gaither Road
Rockville, MD 20850
www.ahrq.gov

Contract No. 290-2007-10055-I

Prepared by:
Tufts Evidence-based Practice Center
Boston, MA

Investigators:
Stanley Ip, M.D., M.S.
Gowri Raman, M.D., M.S.
Thomas W. Concannon, Ph.D.
Sara J. Ratichek, M.A.
Winifred Yu, Ph.D.
Lina Kong Win Chang, B.S.
Ramon Iovin, Ph.D.

AHRQ Publication No. 13-EHC016-EF
February 2013

This report is based on research conducted by the Tufts Evidence-based Practice Center (EPC) under contract to the Agency for Healthcare Research and Quality (AHRQ), Rockville, MD (Contract No. 290-2007-10055-I). The findings and conclusions in this document are those of the author(s), who are responsible for its contents; the findings and conclusions do not necessarily represent the views of AHRQ. Therefore, no statement in this report should be construed as an official position of AHRQ or of the U.S. Department of Health and Human Services.

The information in this report is intended to help health care researchers and funders of research make well-informed decisions in designing and funding research and thereby improve the quality of health care services. This report is not intended to be a substitute for the application of scientific judgment. Anyone who makes decisions concerning the provision of clinical care should consider this report in the same way as any medical research and in conjunction with all other pertinent information, i.e., in the context of available resources and circumstances.

Persons using assistive technology may not be able to fully access information in this report. For assistance contact EffectiveHealthCare@ahrq.hhs.gov.

None of the investigators have any affiliations or financial involvement that conflicts with the material presented in this report.

Suggested citation: Ip S, Raman G, Concannon T, Ratichek SJ, Yu W, Kong Win Chang L, Iovin R. Intravascular Diagnostic Procedures and Imaging Techniques Versus Angiography Alone in Coronary Artery Stenting: Future Research Needs. Future Research Needs Paper No. 25. (Prepared by Tufts Evidence-based Practice Center under Contract No. 290-2007-10055-I.) AHRQ Publication No. 13-EHC016-EF. Rockville, MD: Agency for Healthcare Research and Quality. February 2013. www.effectivehealthcare.ahrq.gov/reports/final.cfm.

Preface

The Agency for Healthcare Research and Quality (AHRQ), through its Evidence-based Practice Centers (EPCs), sponsors the development of evidence reports and technology assessments to assist public- and private-sector organizations in their efforts to improve the quality of health care in the United States. The reports and assessments provide organizations with comprehensive, science-based information on common, costly medical conditions and new health care technologies and strategies. The EPCs systematically review the relevant scientific literature on topics assigned to them by AHRQ and conduct additional analyses when appropriate prior to developing their reports and assessments.

An important part of evidence reports is to not only synthesize the evidence, but also to identify the gaps in evidence that limited the ability to answer the systematic review questions. AHRQ supports EPCs to work with various stakeholders to identify and prioritize the future research that is needed by decisionmakers. This information is provided for researchers and funders of research in these Future Research Needs papers. These papers are made available for public comment and use and may be revised.

AHRQ expects that the EPC evidence reports and technology assessments will inform individual health plans, providers, and purchasers as well as the health care system as a whole by providing important information to help improve health care quality. The evidence reports undergo public comment prior to their release as a final report.

We welcome comments on this Future Research Needs document. They may be sent by mail to the Task Order Officer named below at: Agency for Healthcare Research and Quality, 540 Gaither Road, Rockville, MD 20850, or by email to epc@ahrq.hhs.gov.

Carolyn M. Clancy, M.D.
Director
Agency for Healthcare Research and Quality

Jean Slutsky, P.A., M.S.P.H.
Director, Center for Outcomes and Evidence
Agency for Healthcare Research and Quality

Stephanie Chang, M.D., M.P.H.
Director, EPC Program
Center for Outcomes and Evidence
Agency for Healthcare Research and Quality

Elisabeth U. Kato, M.D., M.R.P.
Task Order Officer
Center for Outcomes and Evidence
Agency for Healthcare Research and Quality

Acknowledgments

The authors gratefully acknowledge the stakeholders for their contributions to this project.

Contributors

J. Matthew Brennan, M.D., M.P.H.
Division of Cardiovascular Disease
Duke University Medical Center
Durham, NC

Marylou Depeiza
Patient representative
Boston, MA

Anton B. Dodek, M.D.
Quality and Consultative Support
Blue Cross Blue Shield of Massachusetts
Boston, MA

Anne Pelikan
Patient representative
Ipswich, MA

Deeb N. Salem, M.D.
Department of Medicine
Tufts University School of Medicine
Boston, MA

Ashwini Sastry, M.D.
Office of Device Evaluation
Interventional Cardiology Devices Branch
Food and Drug Administration
Silver Spring, MD

Jyme Schafer, M.D.
Centers for Medicare and Medicaid Services
Baltimore, MD

Donald S. Shepard, Ph.D.
The Heller School for Social Policy and
    Management
Brandeis University
Waltham, MA

Monvadi B. Srichai-Parsia, M.D., FAHA, FACC
Department of Radiology and Medicine
NYU School of Medicine
New York, NY

Sergio Waxman, M.D.
Tufts University School of Medicine
Boston, MA

Adam Zucker, M.D.
Center for Devices and Radiological Health
Food and Drug Administration
Silver Spring, MD

Intravascular Diagnostic Procedures and Imaging Techniques Versus Angiography Alone in Coronary Artery Stenting: Future Research Needs

Structured Abstract

Background. The optimal use of intravascular diagnostic techniques in patients with coronary artery diseases who are being considered for stenting remains to be defined.

Purpose. Generate prioritized topics for future research on the use of intravascular diagnostic techniques, building on evidence gaps identified in a prior comparative effectiveness review (CER) and following an explicit stakeholder-driven nomination and prioritization process.

Methods. Building on evidence gaps identified in a previous CER on intravascular diagnostic techniques, a preliminary list of future research needs (FRN) was supplemented and refined through input from stakeholders. Stakeholders were asked to rate each proposed priority topic considering the following dimensions in prioritization: (1) importance, (2) desirability of research/avoidance of unnecessary duplication, (3) feasibility, and (4) potential impact. The three topics with the highest number of stakeholder endorsements were identified as the prioritized FRN topics.

Future research needs topics. Two topics (one on the use of intravascular physiologic measurements like fractional flow reserve in treatment decisionmaking before stenting and one on the impact of the use of intravascular imaging diagnostics on stenting) are based directly on evidence gaps identified in the CER. One topic on the added value of intravascular diagnostic techniques in patients for whom there is already a clear clinical and other noninvasive diagnostic indication suggesting the need for revascularization was raised by the stakeholders.

Conclusions. This report identifies three high priority future research needs with regards to intravascular diagnostic techniques, as determined by a stakeholder panel. Both data from pragmatic randomized controlled trials and properly adjusted observational studies could be used to fill the gaps and help address the important clinical questions.

Contents

Executive Summary ES-1

Background 1
   Scope of CER 1
   CER Study Selection and Outcomes of Interest 2
   Findings of the CER 3
   Identification of Evidence Gaps 3
   Analytic Framework 5

Methods 6
   Approach to Evidence Gap Identification 7
      Stakeholder Panel 7
      Identification and Invitation of Individual Stakeholders 8
      Introduction of Process to the Stakeholder Panel 9
      Iterative Process To Identify Future Research Needs Topics 9
   Approach to Prioritization 9
   Approach to Stakeholder Engagement for Prioritization 10
   Approach to Research Question Development and Considerations for Potential
   Research Designs 10

Results 12
   Research Needs 12
      High-Priority Future Research Needs Topic 1 14
      High-Priority Future Research Needs Topic 2 15
      High-Priority Future Research Needs Topic 3 18

Discussion 20

Conclusion 21

References 22

Acronyms and Abbreviations 26

Tables

Table A. Evidence gaps affecting conclusions for the Key Questions ES-3
Table B. Prioritized topics for future research needs in intravascrular diagnostics,
   compared with angiography alone ES-6
Table 1. Evidence gaps inferred from CER findings 4
Table 2. Stakeholders invited 8
Table 3. Prioritized topics for future research needs in intravascular diagnostics, compared
   with angiography alone 13

Figures

Figure A. Analytic framework ES-4
Figure 1. Analytic framework 5
Figure 2. Future research needs process 6

Appendix

Appendix A. Effective Health Care Program Selection Criteria

Executive Summary

Background

Coronary artery disease (CAD), is a narrowing (stenosis) of one or more of the epicardial coronary arteries. It is most commonly due to the buildup of plaque (atherosclerosis), which impedes the ability of these blood vessels to deliver oxygenated blood to the heart muscle (myocardium). Revascularization of the stenotic vessel either by dilatation using a balloon (also known as angioplasty) or by using a bypass venous graft (also known as coronary bypass) are the most common methods to restore blood supply. Percutaneous coronary intervention (PCI) or angioplasty with stent deployment is currently the most commonly performed revascularization procedure for CAD.

PCI has traditionally been based on qualitative and quantitative coronary angiography (visual inspection of the radiocontrast lumenogram and computer-based quantification, respectively), an imaging technique for visualizing the interior of blood vessels. While angiography is the standard technique for anatomic visualization of coronary arteries, it is not without limitations as it does not provide information about what is causing the narrowing or whether the narrowing seriously impedes blood flow. Several adjunctive intravascular diagnostic procedures and imaging techniques (collectively referred to as intravascular diagnostic techniques in this report) have been developed for the purpose of providing more detailed anatomic and hemodynamic information about lesions in coronary arteries. However, whether this additional information improves patient outcomes and whether this improvement outweighs any risks introduced by the additional procedure needs to be considered.

The current Future Research Needs (FRN) project was launched upon the completion of an Agency for Healthcare Research and Quality (AHRQ) comparative effectiveness review (CER) on intravascular diagnostic techniques, and builds on the evidence gaps identified in that review. The CER found 37 studies that directly compared patient outcomes for different techniques. The two techniques that were considered in these studies were fractional flow reserve (FFR) and intravascular ultrasound (IVUS). FFR is a physiologic technique that measures pressure difference using a guide wire across a coronary artery stenosis; it is the ratio between pressure after and pressure before a coronary artery stenosis under conditions of maximum cardiac blood flow (higher ratio suggests less impediment to blood flow across the stenosis). IVUS is an imaging technique that depicts the nature of the atheromatous plaques and the anatomy of the artery wall. All of the studies that aimed to determine which lesions require stenting involved FFR, while most of the studies that looked at optimizing stent placement (i.e., stent size and dilation) involved IVUS. Using criteria based on the AHRQ CER Methods Guide (www.ncbi.nlm.nih.gov/books/NBK47095), we assessed the strength of evidence for major comparisons of interest, as follows:

- There is a moderate strength of evidence (drawn from one randomized controlled trial [RCT] and one nonrandomized study) that the adjunctive use of FFR during stenting, as compared with angiography alone, to decide whether an intermediate coronary lesion (50 to 70% stenosis) requires stenting, can confer a lower risk of composite endpoint of death or myocardial infarction (MI) or of major adverse cardiac event (MACE), decrease procedural costs, and lead to fewer stent implantations. However, these FFR studies also included patients with low risk lesions and lower grades of angina, and excluded left main coronary artery disease and acute MI.

- There is a moderate strength of evidence (drawn from 9 RCTs and 22 nonrandomized studies) that supports no significant difference in mortality and MI, but a significant reduction in restenosis and repeat revascularizations with IVUS-guided stenting compared with stent placement guided by angiography alone. This significant reduction was observed in RCTs, but not observed in nonrandomized comparative studies. Notably, most of the RCTs were conducted before 2000 using previous generation bare-metal stents.
- There is insufficient evidence concerning the use of any intravascular diagnostic techniques immediately after PCI to evaluate the success of stent placement as compared with angiography, or for direct comparisons between intravascular diagnostic techniques.
- There is a moderate strength of evidence (on the basis of one large-sample-size nonrandomized study) that sex, diabetes mellitus status, lesion length and reference diameter, and interaction with IVUS- and angiography-guided stent placement did not show any significant association with individual components of death or MI or the composite outcome of MACE.
- There is insufficient evidence to evaluate the comparative effect of techniques other than FFR and IVUS on outcomes.

The present report describes the development of a stakeholder-prioritized list of research needs for that topic, along with a measured consideration of the advantages and disadvantages of various potential research designs, in order to help researchers and funders develop future research proposals or solicitations.

The evidence gaps identified in the intravascular diagnostic techniques CER are summarized in Table A, organized and labeled by Key Question and PICOD (Population, Intervention, Comparator, Outcome, study Design) category. These gaps limited the conclusions that could be drawn in the original CER, and thus became the initial list of priority topics for the present FRN project. Figure A depicts the analytic framework used to guide the Key Questions for the CER.

Table A. Evidence gaps affecting conclusions for the Key Questions

Key Question	PICO Categories	Evidence Gap
1	Population	**For the comparison between FFR-guided stenting or other intravascular diagnostic techniques and stenting guided by angiography alone:** Because the included studies enrolled a large proportion (>75%) of male patients with lower grades of angina, there is an evidence gap comparing the use of FFR-guided PCI with angiography-guided PCI in female patients and in patients with more serious diseases like LMD or acute MI.
	Intervention	There is an overall evidence gap for this comparison because there were only 3 comparative studies on FFR.
	Comparator	There is an evidence gap comparing patients with low angina score who are potentially eligible to receive aggressive medical therapy instead of PCI to patients who will receive stenting guided by adjunctive FFR, other intravascular diagnostic techniques, or angiography alone.
	Outcome	There is an evidence gap for within 30-day outcomes because the single RCT only reported periprocedural MI, but did not provide data for in-hospital death, repeat revascularizations, or composite endpoint of MACE.
	General evidence gap	There is an overall evidence gap for this comparison because no studies compared the use of other intravascular diagnostic techniques besides FFR and angiography.
2	Population	**For the comparison between IVUS (intravascular ultrasound)-guided stent placement and stenting guided by angiography alone:** The vast majority of included studies enrolled a large proportion (>75%) of male patients and all but one RCT specifically excluded patients with LMD or acute MI. Therefore, there is an evidence gap comparing the use of IVUS-guided PCI with angiography-guided PCI in female patients and in patients with more serious diseases like LMD or acute MI.
	Intervention	There is a lack of IVUS trial data on the influence of operator's choice of balloon size and inflation pressures and their impact on clinical outcomes.
	Comparator	Because only two studies (both RCTs) conducted after year 2000 used the newer and current drug-eluting stents, there is an evidence gap concerning the use of newer types of stents.
	Outcome	There is an evidence gap concerning long-term outcomes since neither RCT reported data on cardiac mortality and few studies reported outcomes greater than 1 year.
	General evidence gap	There is an overall evidence gap for this comparison because no studies compared the use of other intravascular diagnostic techniques besides IVUS and angiography.
3	General evidence gap	**On the impact of using an intravascular diagnostic technique or angiography to evaluate the success of stenting immediately after the procedure:** There is an evidence gap because only two observational studies (both with a high risk for bias) addressed this question.
4	General evidence gap	**Comparing different intravascular diagnostic techniques:** There is an evidence gap because only one observational study with a high risk for bias addressed this question comparing IVUS with FFR.
5	General evidence gap	**Subgroups of interest:** No studies evaluated additional subgroups of interest, including patients with and without diabetes, patients with chronic inflammation (e.g., systemic lupus erythematosus), and patients with atherosclerosis following heart transplantation. There is an evidence gap in terms of lack of reporting of subgroup analyses of patients who underwent intravascular diagnostic-guided PCI compared with angiography-guided PCI and their impact on outcomes.

Abbreviations: FFR = Fractional flow reserve; IVUS = intravascular ultrasound; LMD = left main coronary disease; MACE = major adverse cardiac event; MI = myocardial infarction; PCI = percutaneous coronary intervention; PICO = population, intervention, comparator, outcome; RCT = randomized controlled trial

Figure A. Analytic framework

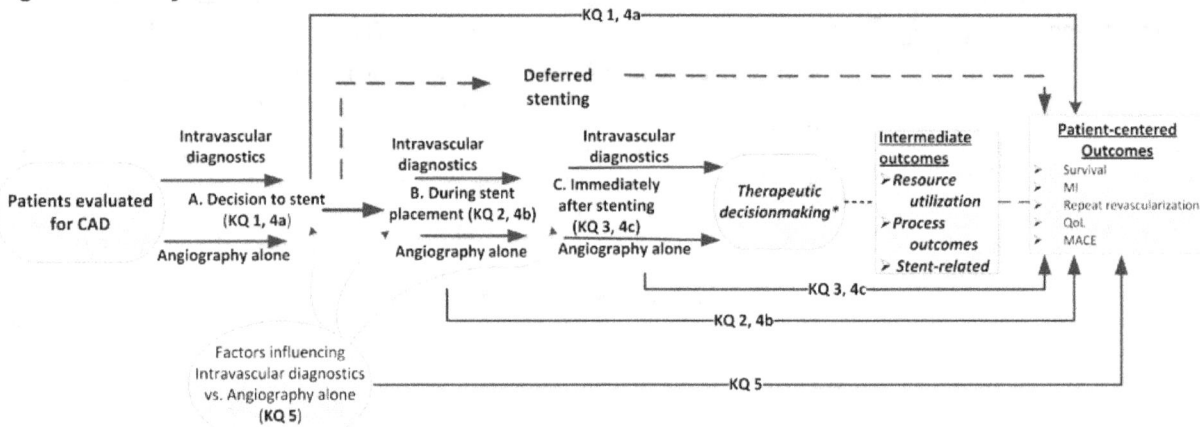

Abbreviations: CAD = coronary artery disease; KQ = Key Question; MACE = major adverse cardiac events; MI = myocardial infarction; QoL = quality of life

Methods

Identifying and Engaging a Stakeholder Panel

We followed a recently developed taxonomy that was designed to aid researchers in the identification, recruitment, and engagement of stakeholders.[1] Based on an a priori categorization of stakeholders according to type, we convened a panel consisting of two patients, four providers, two payers, one policymaker, and one researcher. The stakeholders were provided with the executive summary of the intravascular diagnostics CER and went through a formal orientation process.

Identifying Evidence Gaps and Developing PICOD for Each Gap

As the authors of the intravascular diagnostic techniques CER, we generated the initial list of FRN topics based on the Research Needs section of the report, and then organized the list of evidence gaps according to Key Questionss and PICOD elements. Participating panelists reviewed the preliminary topics and used an iterative process to identify additional FRN topics through webinars and emails.

Criteria for Prioritizing Evidence Gaps

Stakeholders were asked to consider four dimensions of need. These four dimensions are outlined in the Effective Health Care (EHC) Program Selection Criteria and consist of: (1) importance, (2) desirability of research/avoidance of unnecessary duplication, (3) feasibility, and (4) potential impact. The fifth dimension of the EHC program selection criteria, appropriateness, was not evaluated by the stakeholders, as AHRQ had already deemed the topic of intravascular diagnostics to adequately meet this criterion.

Approach to Prioritization

Following two rounds of Webinar discussions and email communication, the topic list was finalized. Stakeholders were asked to rate each of the proposed FRN topics according to the pertinent EHC Program criteria.

Developing Research Questions

We transformed the final list of FRN topics into research questions using standard PICOD criteria. We discussed various alternatives for future research efforts aimed at answering each question, specifically considering the feasibility of addressing the research questions with respect to the study design, potential sample size, the time required, recruitment, and ethical issues.

Results

The FRN identification process led to the nomination of 12 topics (Table B). The three topics where more than 50 percent of the stakeholders had selected them as high priority constitute the highest priority FRN topics. Two topics (one on the use of intravascular physiologic measurements like FFR in treatment decisionmaking before stenting; one on the impact of the use of intravascular imaging diagnostics such as IVUS on stenting) are based directly on evidence gaps identified in the CER. Although the evidence for the topic on intravascular physiologic measurements was rated to be of moderate strength, the stakeholders felt more research was needed for a number of reasons. First, as evidence currently rests primarily on one RCT, there is the possibility that future studies will not support the favorable effect of FFR-guided stenting. Second, given the widespread use of stents (with associated harms and costs) and the well documented variation in practice, any technology that can better target risks and benefits could have a major impact on patient outcomes and healthcare costs. As such it is important to fully explore dimensions beyond what is covered in existing trials.

For the second topic on imaging diagnostics, there is a lack of data on the use of IVUS, as compared with angiography alone, to evaluate placement of newer types of stents including bioabsorbable ones. The third topic on the added value of intravascular diagnostic techniques in patients for whom there is already a clear clinical or other non-invasive diagnostic indication (e.g., a high-risk positive stress perfusion scan, a noninvasive imaging technique that demonstrated large areas of decreased blood flow in the heart) suggesting the need for revascularization was raised by the stakeholders.

Table B. Prioritized topics for future research needs in intravascular diagnostics, compared with angiography alone

Topic*	Topic Questions	Number of Stakeholders Who Think This Is a High-Priority Topic	Mean
Prioritized Future Research Needs Topics			
1	What is the impact on clinical outcomes of a treatment decision (medical therapy, stent, or bypass) made on the basis of the adjunctive use of intravascular physiologic diagnostics, as compared with angiography alone?	7	4.67
2	In patients in whom there is already a precatheterization indication for stenting, what is the impact on stenting parameters (e.g., which lesion to stent, type of stent, stent length) and clinical outcomes of the use versus non-use of intravascular diagnostics?	6	4.44
3	Once the decision has been made to place a stent, what is the impact on clinical outcomes of the adjunctive use of intravascular imaging diagnostics, such as IVUS or OCT, in stent placement and stent optimization, as compared with angiography alone?	5	4.22
Other Topics			
4	What is the impact on clinical outcomes of a treatment decision (medical therapy, stent, or bypass) made on the basis of the adjunctive use of intravascular imaging diagnostics, such as IVUS or OCT, as compared with angiography alone?	4	4.11
5	What is the impact of baseline characteristics (e.g., sex, age, co-morbidities, type of lesions, severity of disease) on clinical outcomes when using intravascular diagnostics during coronary stenting, as compared with angiography alone?	4	4.00
6	What is the impact on clinical outcomes of operator experience, as measured by the number of completed procedures in using intravascular diagnostics?	4	3.78
7	What is the impact on clinical outcomes of a treatment decision (medical therapy, stent, or bypass) made on the basis of the adjunctive use of intravascular physiologic diagnostics, as compared with other intravascular diagnostics?	3	3.67
8	What is the impact on clinical outcomes of a treatment decision (medical therapy, stent, or bypass) made on the basis of the adjunctive use of intravascular imaging diagnostics, such as IVUS or OCT, as compared with FFR?	3	3.67
9	What adverse events and complications have been associated with the use of intravascular diagnostic procedures for coronary stenting, as compared with angiography alone?	2	3.44
10	Once the decision has been made to place a stent, what is the impact on clinical outcomes of the adjunctive use of intravascular imaging diagnostics, such as IVUS or OCT, during stenting and stent optimization, as compared with other intravascular diagnostics such as FFR?	2	3.22
11	What is the impact on clinical outcomes of the adjunctive use of new and on-the-horizon or hybrid intravascular diagnostics, as compared with angiography alone or other established techniques such as FFR or IVUS?	2	3.33
12	What is the impact on therapeutic decisionmaking and clinical outcomes of the use of intravascular diagnostics in patients who were discovered to have no evidence of coronary artery disease by angiography (such as in patients examined due to intense coronary vasospasm)?	2	3

Abbreviations: FFR = fractional flow reserve; IVUS = intravascular ultrasound; OCT = optical coherence tomography
*Prioritized topics (1–12) are listed in the order they were prioritized by the stakeholder panel.

In research comparing clinical interventions, RCTs are the optimal study design, but ethical and feasibility concerns can make this methodology difficult or impossible to justify. An RCT to address the first topic—the adjunctive use of intravascular diagnostic techniques like FFR—for instance, would be difficult to conduct as FFR-guided PCI is already becoming the standard of care in patients with borderline and intermediate lesions. Therefore, to address this topic, an observational design is a feasible alternative. An observational study could be used to compare the outcomes of treatment decision made on the basis of FFR versus no FFR, if established methodological approaches like matching, propensity score analyses, and other techniques, are used to adjust for baseline differences between groups.

For the second topic on the adjunctive use of intravascular diagnostic techniques in patients with a clear clinical or other noninvasive diagnostic indication suggesting the potential need for revascularization (stenting or coronary bypass graft), because IVUS and FFR serve different purposes (IVUS helps to optimize stenting parameters like stent lengths, stent inflation pressure, and others; FFR helps to define the need for stenting and which lesions to stent), we propose different study designs depending on the particular intravascular diagnostic modality.

For IVUS, we propose a pragmatic trial of use versus nonuse of IVUS to examine the impact on stenting parameters and clinical outcomes. For FFR, an RCT comparing the use versus nonuse of FFR-guided angiography in patients with high-risk positive stress test may be difficult to conduct as FFR-guided PCI is fast becoming the standard of care. Therefore, an observational study design is recommended for FFR.

Similarly, in those with a negative stress test and the presence of classic symptom complex, as providers may use IVUS and/or FFR to help make a determination on the need for stenting, it would also be difficult to recruit providers and patients for an RCT in this setting. In this setting, we therefore propose a prospective observational study design, using a combination of catheterization registry data that are derived directly from electronic health records, linked with Medicare claims and state mortality records. Treatment assignment would be non-random, but statistical techniques could be used to adjust for potential confounding from treatment selection.

For the third topic on how the adjunctive use of intravascular diagnostic techniques affects stenting, a pragmatic RCT comparing the use of intravascular diagnostics versus angiography alone on stenting parameters and clinical outcomes would help to fill in the evidence gaps. Observational studies may also help to fill in the gap but existing registries like the CathPCI database do not have enough details on stenting parameters to help address these questions (e.g., the impact of intravascular diagnostic techniques on stent "optimization" and clinical outcomes). A novel module could be implemented in the CathPCI registry to collect additional IVUS parameters and additional stenting parameters. These data could be used to assess how IVUS influenced the procedure.

Discussion

The use of intravascular diagnostics in patients being considered for percutaneous coronary artery stenting is a highly technical topic and requires considerable domain knowledge to appreciate how these adjunctive diagnostics aid traditional coronary artery catheterization and stenting. Added to this difficulty is the challenge of defining optimal stent placement; this concept has permeated the clinical community but standards have not been established.

To identify priority future research needs we sought and successfully incorporated insight from clinical experts as well as from insurance, hospital, patient and policy experts. Additionally, we have asked domain experts to review the description of the technical details concerning these diagnostic devices, to assure that it is faithful to the complex clinical details of intravascular diagnostic technology as applied to cardiovascular disease.

Conclusions

This report identifies three high-priority future research needs with regards to intravascular diagnostic techniques, as determined by a stakeholder panel. They are:

1. What is the impact on clinical outcomes of a treatment decision (medical therapy, stent, or bypass) made on the basis of the adjunctive use of intravascular physiologic diagnostics, as compared with angiography alone?

2. In patients in whom there is already a clear clinical and other non-invasive diagnostic indication suggesting the need for revascularization (stenting or coronary artery bypass graft), what is the impact on stenting parameters (e.g., which lesion to stent, type of stent, stent length) and clinical outcomes of the use versus non-use of intravascular diagnostics in those undergoing stenting?

3. Once the decision has been made to place a stent, what is the impact on clinical outcomes of the adjunctive use of intravascular imaging diagnostics, such as IVUS or OCT, in stent placement and stent optimization, as compared with angiography alone?

In summary, both data from pragmatic randomized controlled trials and properly adjusted observational studies could be used to fill in these gaps and help address these important clinical questions.

Background

Coronary artery disease (CAD), is a narrowing (stenosis) of one or more of the epicardial coronary arteries. It is most commonly due to the buildup of plaque (atherosclerosis), which impedes the ability of these blood vessels to deliver oxygenated blood to the heart muscle (myocardium). Revascularization of the stenotic vessel either by dilatation using a balloon (also known as angioplasty) or by using a bypass venous graft (also known as coronary bypass) are the most common methods to restore blood supply. Percutaneous coronary intervention (PCI) or angioplasty with stent deployment is currently the most commonly performed revascularization procedure for CAD.

PCI has traditionally been based on qualitative and quantitative coronary angiography (visual inspection of the radiocontrast lumenogram and computer-based quantification, respectively), an imaging technique for visualizing the interior of blood vessels. While angiography is the standard technique for anatomic visualization of coronary arteries, it is not without limitations as it does not provide information about what is causing the narrowing or whether the narrowing seriously impedes blood flow. Several adjunctive intravascular diagnostic procedures and imaging techniques (collectively referred to as intravascular diagnostic techniques in this report) have been developed for the purpose of providing more detailed anatomic and hemodynamic information about lesions in coronary arteries. However, whether this additional information improves patient outcomes and whether this improvement outweighs any risks introduced by the additional procedure has yet to be determined.

The current Future Research Needs (FRN) project was launched upon the completion of an Agency for Healthcare Research and Quality (AHRQ) comparative effectiveness review (CER) on intravascular diagnostic techniques,[2] and builds on the evidence gaps identified in that review. The present report describes the development of a stakeholder-prioritized list of research needs for that topic, along with a measured consideration of the advantages and disadvantages of various potential research designs, in order to help researchers and funders develop future research proposals or solicitations.

Scope of CER

The 2013 CER upon which the current FRN report is based, "Intravascular Diagnostic Procedures and Imaging Techniques Versus Angiography Alone," was sponsored by the Agency for Healthcare Research and Quality and conducted by the Tufts Evidence-based Practice Center (EPC).[2] It reviewed pertinent publications through May 2012 and addressed five Key Questions:

Key Question 1. In patients with CAD, what is the impact of using an intravascular diagnostic technique and angiography in deciding whether a coronary lesion requires stenting—when compared with angiography alone—on therapeutic decisionmaking, and intermediate and patient-centered outcomes?

Key Question 2. For patients undergoing PCI, what is the impact of using an intravascular diagnostic technique and angiography to guide the stenting procedure (either immediately prior to or during the procedure)—when compared with angiography-guided stenting—on therapeutic decisionmaking, and intermediate and patient-centered outcomes?

Key Question 3. For patients having just undergone a PCI with stenting, what is the impact of using an intravascular diagnostic technique and angiography to evaluate the success of stenting immediately after the procedure—when compared with angiography alone—on therapeutic decisionmaking, and intermediate and patient-centered outcomes?

Key Question 4. How do different intravascular diagnostic techniques compare with each other in their effects on therapeutic decisionmaking, and intermediate and patient-centered outcomes?
  a. During diagnostic coronary angiography for the evaluation of the presence/extent of CAD and the potential need for coronary intervention?
  b. During PCI to guide stenting?
  c. Immediately after PCI to evaluate the success of stenting?

Key Question 5. What factors (e.g., patient/physician characteristics, availability of prior noninvasive testing, type of PCI performed) influence the effect of intravascular diagnostic technique and angiography—when compared with angiography (or among different intravascular diagnostic technique techniques)—on therapeutic decisionmaking, and intermediate and patient-centered outcomes?
  a. During coronary angiography for the evaluation of the presence/extent of CAD and the potential need for coronary stenting
  b. During PCI to guide stenting
  c. Immediately after PCI to evaluate the success of stenting

Therapeutic decisionmaking outcomes outlined in the Key Questions were defined as follows:
  • **Key Question 1**: In patients with CAD, the change in the number of hemodynamically significant lesions after the application of intravascular diagnostic, and the change in the decision about an interventional therapy (e.g., if stenting is needed) after the application of intravascular diagnostic technique
  • **Key Question 2**: During PCI, the change in the type of stent or number of stents or length of stent after the application of intravascular diagnostic technique
  • **Key Question 3**: Immediately after PCI, the need for additional stenting modifications

CER Study Selection and Outcomes of Interest

Each question had specific criteria for study inclusion based on the PICOD (Population, Intervention, Comparator, Outcomes, and Design) categorization. We included studies conducted in adults (≥18 years of age) with CAD who were being considered for PCI with stenting. All forms of CAD presentation were included. Coronary angiography was the comparison of interest for Key Questions 1, 2, 3, and 5. For Key Question 4, head-to-head comparisons of two or more intravascular diagnostic techniques were examined. For Key Question 5, the modifiers of treatment effect included patient/physician characteristics, availability of prior noninvasive testing, and the type of PCI performed.

Outcomes of interest included therapeutic decisionmaking; patient-centered outcomes (e.g., mortality and cardiovascular events); intermediate outcomes (e.g., minimal lumen diameter, percent diameter stenosis, and stent-related outcomes [e.g. restenosis, stent thrombosis]). They were further categorized on the basis of timing of followup: in-hospital outcomes, short-term outcomes (discharge to 30 days), medium-term outcomes (>30 days to 1 year), and long-term outcomes (>1 year).

Findings of the CER

In total, 37 unique studies (in 41 published articles) met eligibility criteria.[3-43] The two most commonly evaluated intravascular diagnostic techniques were intravascular ultrasound (IVUS) and fractional flow reserve (FFR). Findings are as follows:

- For Key Question 1, there was moderate evidence (drawn from one randomized controlled trial [RCT] and one nonrandomized study) that the use of FFR in deciding whether a coronary lesion requires stenting, as compared with angiography-guided stenting, can confer a lower risk of composite endpoint of death or myocardial infarction (MI) or of major adverse cardiac events (MACE), decrease procedural costs, and lead to fewer stents implantations.

- For Key Question 2, there was moderate evidence (drawn from 9 RCTs and 22 nonrandomized studies) that fails to support a statistically significant difference in most clinical and intermediate outcomes between IVUS-guided and angiography-guided stenting patient groups.[a]

- For Key Questions 3 and 4, there was insufficient evidence (two nonrandomized studies of small sample size, rated as being at high risk of bias) concerning the use of intravascular diagnostic techniques immediately after PCI to evaluate the success of stenting as compared with angiography-guided stenting, or for direct comparisons between intravascular diagnostic techniques.

- For Key Question 5, there was moderate evidence (on the basis of one nonrandomized study of 9,070 patients) that any interaction of sex, diabetes mellitus status, lesion length or reference diameter with IVUS- and angiography-guided stenting did not have significant association with individual components or composite outcome of MACE. With the exception of IVUS and FFR, there was insufficient evidence to evaluate the comparative effect of any other intravascular diagnostic techniques on the outcomes of interest.

Identification of Evidence Gaps

The current FRN project was undertaken in order to address the evidence gaps in the literature with regards to intravascular diagnostic techniques and their comparative effectiveness, identified during the synthesis of the aforementioned CER. Table 1 summarizes the evidence gaps identified in our review of intravascular diagnostic techniques (listed in no particular order).

---

[a]For followup up to 1 year in randomized trials, a lower risk of repeat revascularization (summary relative risk: 0.70; 95% CI [0.51, 0.97]) but a higher risk of mortality (summary relative risk: 1.84; 95% CI [0.88, 3.85]) in the IVUS group was observed, compared with the angiography group. Any observed significant differences in intermediate outcomes were small and inconsistent.

Table 1. Evidence gaps inferred from CER findings

Key Question	PICO Categories	Evidence Gap
1	Population	**For the comparison between FFR-guided stenting or other intravascular diagnostic techniques and stenting guided by angiography alone:** Because the included studies enrolled a large proportion (>75%) of male patients with lower grades of angina, there is an evidence gap comparing the use of FFR-guided with angiography-guided PCI in female patients and in patients with more serious diseases like LMD or acute MI.
	Intervention	There is an overall evidence gap for this comparison because there were only 3 comparative studies on FFR.
	Comparator	There is an evidence gap comparing patients with low angina score who are potentially eligible to receive aggressive medical therapy instead of PCI to patients who will receive stenting guided by adjunctive FFR, other intravascular diagnostic techniques, or angiography alone.
	Outcome	There is an evidence gap for within 30-day outcomes because the single RCT only reported periprocedural MI, but did not provide data for in-hospital death, repeat revascularization, or MACE.
	General evidence gap	There is an overall evidence gap for this comparison because no studies compared the use of other intravascular diagnostic techniques besides FFR and angiography.
2	Population	**For the comparison between IVUS-guided stent placement and stenting guided by angiography alone:** The vast majority of included studies enrolled a large proportion (>75%) of male patients and all but one RCT specifically excluded patients with LMD or acute MI. Therefore, there is an evidence gap comparing the use of IVUS-guided with angiography-guided PCI in female patients and in patients with more serious diseases like LMD or acute MI.
	Intervention	There is a lack of IVUS trial data on the influence of operator's choice of balloon size and inflation pressures and their impact on clinical outcomes.
	Comparator	Because only two studies (both RCTs) conducted after year 2000 used the newer and current drug eluting stents, there is an evidence gap concerning the use of newer types of stents.
	Outcome	There is an evidence gap concerning long-term outcomes since neither RCT reported data on cardiac mortality and few studies reported outcomes greater than 1 year.
	General evidence gap	There is an overall evidence gap for this comparison because no studies compared the use of other intravascular diagnostic techniques besides IVUS and angiography.
3	General evidence gap	**On the impact of using an intravascular diagnostic technique and angiography to evaluate the success of stenting immediately after the procedure:** There is an evidence gap because only two observational studies and with high risk of bias reported on this comparison.
4	General evidence gap	**Comparing different intravascular diagnostic techniques:** There is an evidence gap because only one observational study and with high risk of bias reported on this comparison (IVUS vs. FFR).
5	General evidence gap	**Subgroups of interest:** No studies evaluated additional subgroups of interest, including patients with and without diabetes, patients with chronic inflammation (e.g., systemic lupus erythematosus), and patients with atherosclerosis following heart transplantation. There is an evidence gap in terms of lack of reporting of subgroup analyses of patients who underwent intravascular diagnostic-guided PCI compared with angiography-guided PCI and their impact on outcomes.

Abbreviations: FFR = Fractional flow reserve; IVUS = intravascular ultrasound; LMD = left main disease; MACE = major adverse cardiac event; MI = myocardial infarction; PCI = percutaneous coronary intervention; PICO = population, intervention, comparator, outcome; RCT = randomized controlled trial

Analytic Framework

The analytic framework (Figure 1) depicts the logical interconnection of all five Key Questions addressed by the CER. It maps the Key Questions within the context of the populations of interest, the interventions, comparator, and the outcomes of interest, and the chain of reasoning that the evidence must support to link the interventions to improved health outcomes. The figure illustrates how the additional application of intravascular diagnostic techniques (compared with angiography alone) may aid treatment decisionmaking during diagnostic angiography (A in the figure), allow procedure optimization during PCI (B), and assessment of immediate results in patients undergoing PCI to decide the need for additional procedures (C), and improve short-term (in hospital or discharge to 30 days), medium-term (≥30 days to 1 year), and long-term (>1 year) outcomes. Angiography alone is the comparator for Key Questions 1–3. For Key Question 4, the comparator is a different intravascular diagnostic technique from the index intravascular diagnostic technique of interest (head-to-head comparisons of intravascular diagnostic techniques). For Key Question 5, potential effect modifiers of treatment effects were examined, for both comparisons between angiography with and without intravascular diagnostic technique and comparisons of two or more intravascular diagnostic techniques. For Key Question 5, the modifiers of treatment effect included patient/physician characteristics, availability of prior noninvasive testing, and the type of PCI performed.

Figure 1. Analytic framework

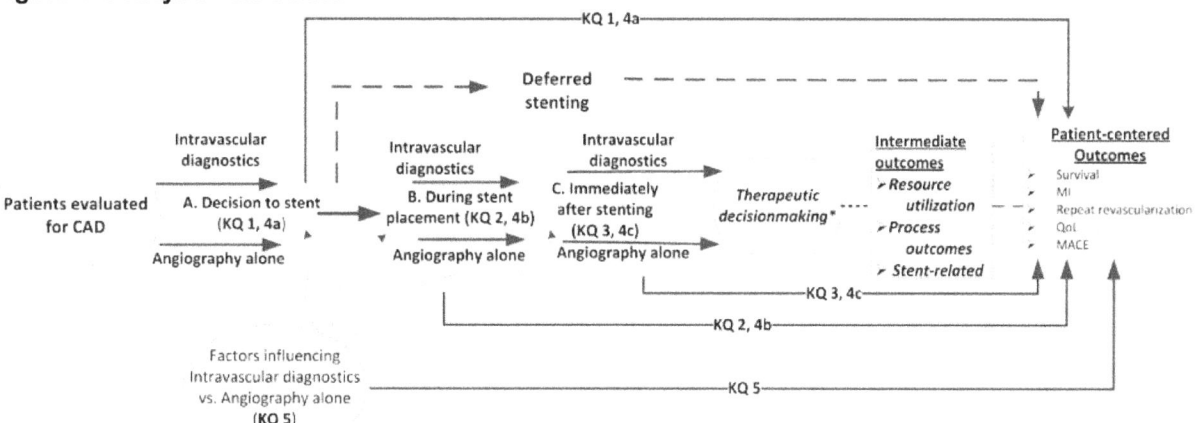

Abbreviations: CAD = coronary artery disease; KQ = Key Question; MACE = major adverse cardiac events; MI = myocardial infarction; QoL = quality of life

Methods

Figure 2 is a flow chart depicting the process for the future research needs project, from invitation of stakeholders and dissemination of background materials through topic nomination and ranking (before, during, and after two Webinars), and development of research protocols for the final lists of future research needs topics. Details for each of the step are described below.

Figure 2. Future research needs process

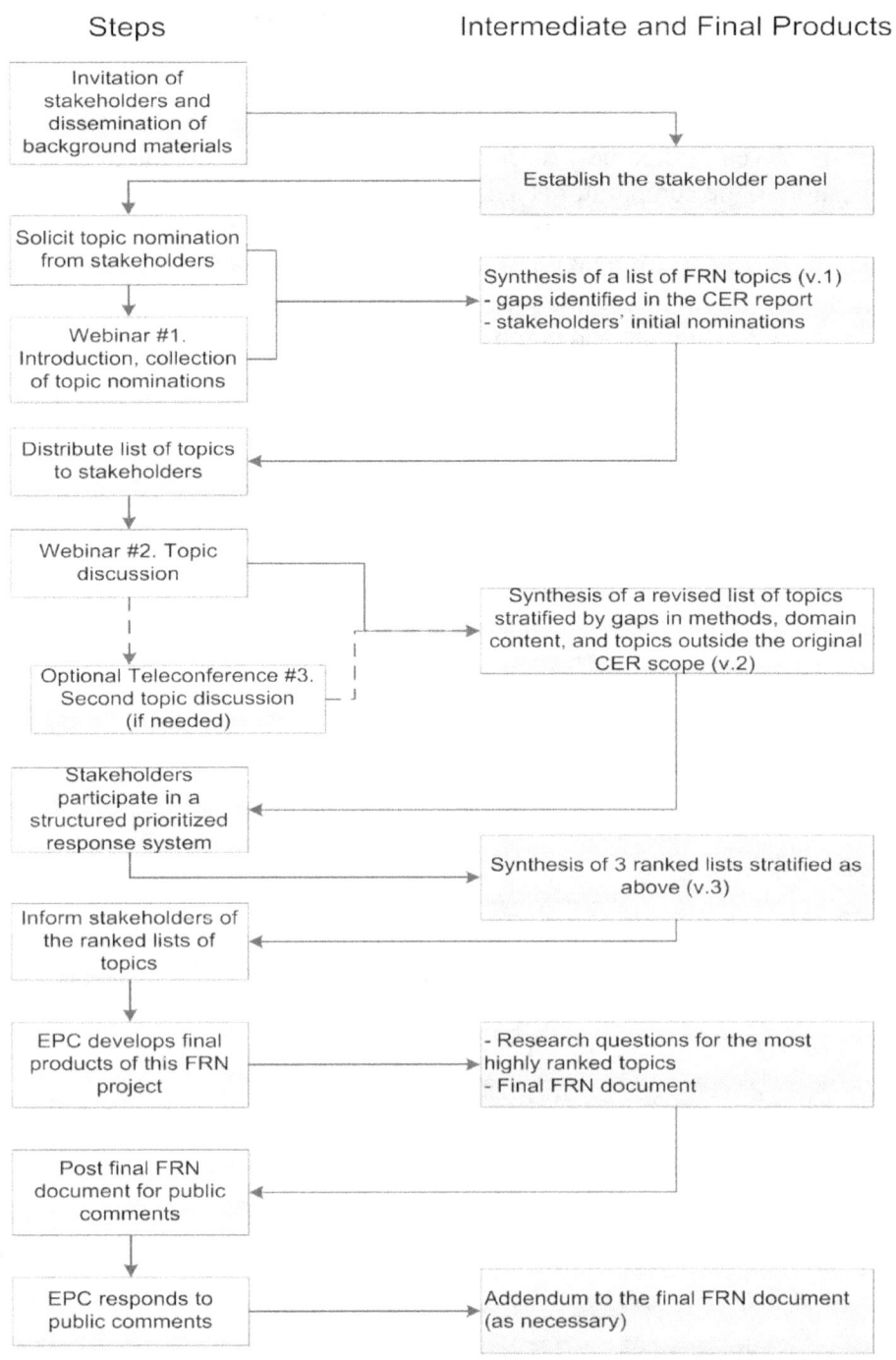

Abbreviations: CER = comparative effectiveness review; EPC = evidence-based practice center; FRN = future research needs

Approach to Evidence Gap Identification

We used an iterative process with a stakeholder panel to identify future research needs topics for prioritization. Based on the evidence gaps identified in the original CER (Table 1), we generated an initial list of FRN topics and then solicited additional topics from the stakeholder panel through teleconferences and emails. To make sure that we are not recommending new trials that are already being conducted elsewhere, on August 31, 2012, we searched ClinicalTrials.gov to find ongoing or recently completed trials relevant to the topic. Three randomized trials were identified.[b]

Stakeholder Panel

We have adapted a Tufts-developed model of stakeholder engagement to identify individuals from seven stakeholder categories. This model was designed to build a panel representing the full range of stakeholders who may use research evidence in health care and public health decisionmaking.

1. **Patients and the Public.** This group represents current and potential consumers of patient-centered healthcare and population-focused public health. This group also includes caregivers, family members, and patient advocacy organizations, all of whom address the interests of consumers.
2. **Providers.** This group includes individuals (e.g., nurses, physicians, and other providers of care and support services) as well as organizations (e.g., hospitals, clinics, community health centers, community based organizations, pharmacies, emergency medical services (EMS) agencies, skilled nursing facilities) that provide care to patients and populations.
3. **Purchasers.** This group includes employers, the self-insured, government, and other entities responsible for underwriting the costs of health care.
4. **Payers.** This group represents insurers, Medicare and Medicaid, individuals with deductibles, and others responsible for reimbursement for interventions and episodes of care.
5. **Product Makers.** This group includes pharmaceutical and medical device manufacturers.
6. **Policymakers.** This group includes organizations such as the White House, Department of Health and Human Services, Congress, states, professional associations, and intermediary groups that collate and distribute information to policymakers.
7. **Principal investigators, researchers, and research funders.** Individuals representing these categories may wear several hats and may be responsible for different types of decisions. For example, some health care purchasers are also

---

[b]The AVIO (NCT00936169) is a completed study from Italy, comparing IVUS versus angiography alone optimization of the use of drug-eluting stents. The results have not been published.

The FAVOR (NCT01175863) is an ongoing randomized trial being conducted in South Korea comparing the effectiveness of FFR-guided versus IVUS-guided PCI for the treatment of intermediate coronary lesions. The primary outcome of this trial is MACE; secondary outcomes are the individual components of MACE. Patients will be followed clinically for up to 2 years. This trial is expected to enroll 1400 patients and will be completed by January 2014.

The DEFER-DES (NCT00592228) was a randomized controlled trial from South Korea, comparing FFR-guided with angiography alone-guided stenting using drug-eluting stents in patients with intermediate coronary lesions. It has since been terminated owing to slow enrollment.

payers, and conversely some payers also provide care. Patients and their advocates may be providers or employers with policymaking responsibilities, and so on. In addition, each of these seven stakeholder types may be focused on applying research evidence at the patient- or population level. Patient-level decisions included questions regarding the best treatment for a given patient at a given time. Population-level decisions included questions regarding the optimal services, resources, policies, and alternatives for groups of patients and other communities connected by practice setting, geography, clinical domain, or other means. To be patient-centered, decisions made about groups of patients must recognize both the diversity of needs across populations and the heterogeneity of individuals within populations.

Because a future research needs project is intended to rank research questions by priority, product makers (i.e., manufacturers of intravascular diagnostic technology) were considered to be in potential conflict of interest. They were therefore restricted to participation in the topic nomination process but not in topic refinement or prioritization. Additionally, purchasers were considered to share the same perspective on this topic as would payers, and therefore were not invited to participate as a distinct group on the panel.

Identification and Invitation of Individual Stakeholders

As part of the protocol development, we created an a priori target number of stakeholders representing each group in our proposed panel (Table 2), attempting to create a balance across stakeholder categories, and seeking to cover a range of technical and personal expertise in the group as a whole. We used these targets to identify individuals to serve on our panel through several means. We began by inviting individuals who have previously served in advisory roles for the EPC's intravascular diagnostic techniques CER. In addition, EPC team members were asked to identify professional contacts that could help us reach the targets for each of the target groups on the panel. Finally, we conducted searches on google.com and MEDLINE® to identify active intravascular diagnostic technique researchers for the provider and principal investigator categories.

An invitation letter was sent to individuals representing each of the final six target groups, and names were added to assemble a representative panel of nine nongovernment stakeholders plus two government stakeholders. All stakeholders completed a standard disclosure of interest form. Again, device makers ("product makers" in the 7Ps taxonomy) were invited to propose topics; they were not invited to participate in refinement or prioritization.

Table 2. Stakeholders invited

Category	Subcategory	Number of Stakeholders
Patients and the public	Current patients	2
Providers	Clinicians – interventional cardiologist	5
	Clinicians – noninterventional cardiologist	
	Clinicians – nurse practitioner or physician assistant	
	Hospital administrator	
Payers	Private insurer	2
	Medicare	
Policymakers	FDA (Food and Drug Administration) devices group	1
Principal investigators/researchers	Health services	1
TOTAL		11

Introduction of Process to the Stakeholder Panel

Along with an invitation letter, we distributed pertinent portions of the executive summary and the "Future Research" section of the original CER draft together with the protocol to the invited stakeholders. The original Key Questions, summary of evidence table, and the implications sections were highlighted in the executive summary. The purpose of the FRN project and the expectations for input from the stakeholders were outlined clearly in the invitation letter.

Soon after populating the panel, to accommodate everyone's schedule[c], we conducted a first round of webinars with different stakeholders over a one week period to explain the purpose and process of the FRN topic development process and to review research gaps in intravascular diagnostic technology. For each nominated topic, stakeholders were also asked to provide a brief rationale to explain why they consider the topic to be a potential priority. When time permitted, we asked stakeholders to briefly describe related topics of interest.

Iterative Process To Identify Future Research Needs Topics

Based on the input from the first round of webinars, we reorganize the topic nomination document into separate topics based both on evidence gaps and additional topics suggested by the stakeholders. We also collated all the stakeholders' comments into their respective topics and distributed this document so everyone can be informed on what each other has opined. A second round of webinars was held to allow stakeholders to voice further opinions about the nominated topics. Stakeholders were also encouraged to provide comments and feedback by email. We prepared minutes of calls and circulated to all participants.

The revisions to the document with the list of FRN topics were based on the discussions and continued on an iterative process.

Approach to Prioritization

Stakeholders were asked to consider four dimensions of need related to the proposed topic. These four dimensions are drawn from the Effective Health Care (EHC) Program Selection Criteria (Appendix A). These dimensions and EHC program guidance were described in detail in the lead up to submission, discussion, and selection of FRN topics. They are:

- Importance
- Desirability of Research/Duplication
- Feasibility
- Potential Impact

A fifth dimension of the Selection Criteria, appropriateness, was not evaluated by the stakeholders, as AHRQ already deemed the topic of intravascular diagnostics to adequately meet this criterion. The EHC Program guidance on these criteria was explained in detail at each webinar encounter with the stakeholders. Please see Appendix A for a more complete description of AHRQ's EHC Program Selection Criteria.

---

[c]We also offered one-on-one conferences (e.g., patients only) on an as needed basis.

Approach to Stakeholder Engagement for Prioritization

With a final list of potential topics, stakeholders were asked to consider the previously mentioned four dimensions of need for each FRN topic by filling in a web form to evaluate each of the 12 nominated topics Stakeholders evaluated each topic as "low priority," "low to intermediate priority," "intermediate priority," "intermediate to high priority," or "high priority."

The EPC ranked the FRN topics based on stakeholder responses to the survey. A count of the topics receiving a "high priority" mention was computed as well as the mean average score for all the topics. Three topics received high priority by more than half of those who participated. These three topics' research needs were further refined.

Approach to Research Question Development and Considerations for Potential Research Designs

The EPC transformed the final list of FRN topics into answerable research questions using standard "PICOD" criteria (Population, Intervention, Comparator, Outcomes, study Design). When necessary, two or more alternative PICOD-based research proposals were offered, and the EPC discussed and described the pros and cons of these alternatives. The EPC specifically considered the feasibility of the research questions, focusing on potential sample size, time, and recruitment issues.

To determine candidate study designs, study feasibility, and sample size calculations, we followed the structure laid out in "Future Research Needs for the Comparison of Percutaneous Coronary Interventions with Bypass Graft Surgery in Nonacute Coronary Artery Disease," written by our EPC (Tufts) as an example FRN document.[d]

Briefly: Candidate study designs will differ across types of research needs. Effectiveness or efficacy of treatments can be most definitively addressed in randomized trials, and secondarily in well-conducted nonrandomized comparative observational studies. In contrast, eliciting patient preferences can be meaningfully performed with nonexperimental designs (for example, in a survey). Furthermore, observational studies may be most appropriate to enhance generalizability and determine effectiveness, as opposed to efficacy alone. Each final FRN topic was assessed as to the context of the research question. A determination was made as to whether evaluation of efficacy or effectiveness is of greater need. This informed the choice of study design. Regardless of study design, a full set of PICO criteria (population, intervention, comparator, outcomes) was proposed.

Studies that do not require new data collection are in principle feasible, provided that access to existing data can be agreed upon or has already been granted. Analysis of an existing registry, standard meta-analysis, or meta-analysis of individual patient data can be conducted in a limited timeframe. The feasibility of such studies, generally, does not depend on the desired sample size. The feasibility of trials (or other studies requiring collection of primary data) may not be feasible if it were too expensive or complex to conduct, if it would require too long a followup, or if it would rely on information or data that is not yet available or would be difficult to obtain. When randomized trials were deemed to be the most appropriate study design to address an FRN topic,

---

[d]Trikalinos TA, Dahabreh IJ, Wong J, Rao M. Future Research Needs for the Comparison of Percutaneous Coronary Interventions with Bypass Graft Surgery in Nonacute Coronary Artery Disease: Identification of Future Research Needs from Comparative Effectiveness Review No. 9 [Internet]. Rockville (MD): Agency for Healthcare Research and Quality (US); 2010 Sep. http://effectivehealthcare.ahrq.gov/index.cfm/search-for-guides-reviews-and-reports/?pageaction= displayproduct&productid=522.

we performed sample size calculations using standard formulae for a two-sided chi-squared test at the 0.05 level of significance. We also estimated the true relative effect between intervention and control. We assumed an allocation ratio of 1:1, no loss to followup, no crossover between treatments, and no sequential monitoring.

As needed, the EPC consulted with individual stakeholders for assistance in making decisions regarding appropriate study designs.

Results

Research Needs

Of 11 stakeholders who were invited, 10 participated in the teleconferences, and 9 participated in the prioritization process. The FRN identification process led to the nomination of 12 topics (Table 3). The three topics with the highest number of stakeholder endorsements constitute the highest priority FRN topics. Two topics (one on the use of intravascular physiologic measurements like FFR in treatment decisionmaking before stenting; one on the impact of the use of intravascular imaging diagnostics on stenting) are based directly on evidence gaps identified in the CER. These two topics are of interest because FFR and IVUS have not been thoroughly studied. There is only one trial comparing FFR with angiography alone to assess the use of FFR to help determine which patients should receive stents. Similarly, there is a lack of data on the use of IVUS, as compared with angiography alone, to evaluate placement of newer types of stents including bioabsorbable ones. The third topic on the added value of intravascular diagnostic techniques in patients for whom there is already a clear clinical or other noninvasive diagnostic indicator (e.g., a high-risk positive stress perfusion scan, a noninvasive imaging technique that demonstrated large areas of decreased blood flow in the heart) for the potential need for revascularization was raised by the stakeholders.

Table 3. Prioritized topics for future research needs in intravascular diagnostics, compared with angiography alone

Topic*	Topic Questions	Number of Stakeholders Who Think This Is a High-Priority Topic	Mean
	Prioritized Future Research Needs Topics		
1	What is the impact on clinical outcomes of a treatment decision (medical therapy, stent, or bypass) made on the basis of the adjunctive use of intravascular physiologic diagnostics, as compared with angiography alone?	7	4.67
2	In patients in whom there is already a precatheterization indication for stenting, what is the impact on stenting parameters (e.g., which lesion to stent, type of stent, stent length) and clinical outcomes of the use versus non-use of intravascular diagnostics?	6	4.44
3	Once the decision has been made to place a stent, what is the impact on clinical outcomes of the adjunctive use of intravascular imaging diagnostics, such as IVUS or OCT, in stent placement and stent optimization, as compared with angiography alone?	5	4.22
	Other Topics		
4	What is the impact on clinical outcomes of a treatment decision (medical therapy, stent, or bypass) made on the basis of the adjunctive use of intravascular imaging diagnostics, such as IVUS or OCT, as compared with angiography alone?	4	4.11
5	What is the impact on clinical outcomes of operator experience, as measured by the number of completed procedures in using intravascular diagnostics?	4	3.78
6	What is the impact of baseline characteristics (e.g., sex, age, co-morbidities, type of lesions, severity of disease) on clinical outcomes when using intravascular diagnostics during coronary stenting, as compared with angiography alone?	4	4.00
7	What is the impact on clinical outcomes of a treatment decision (medical therapy, stent, or bypass) made on the basis of the adjunctive use of intravascular physiologic diagnostics, as compared with other intravascular diagnostics?	3	3.67
8	What is the impact on clinical outcomes of a treatment decision (medical therapy, stent, or bypass) made on the basis of the adjunctive use of intravascular imaging diagnostics, such as IVUS or OCT, as compared with FFR?	3	3.67
9	What adverse events and complications have been associated with the use of intravascular diagnostic procedures for coronary stenting, as compared with angiography alone?	2	3.44
10	Once the decision has been made to place a stent, what is the impact on clinical outcomes of the adjunctive use of intravascular imaging diagnostics, such as IVUS or OCT, during stenting and stent optimization, as compared with other intravascular diagnostics such as FFR?	2	3.22
11	What is the impact on clinical outcomes of the adjunctive use of new and on-the-horizon or hybrid intravascular diagnostics, as compared with angiography alone or other established techniques such as FFR or IVUS?	2	3.33
12	What is the impact on therapeutic decisionmaking and clinical outcomes of the use of intravascular diagnostics in patients who were discovered to have no evidence of coronary artery disease by angiography (such as in patients examined due to intense coronary vasospasm)?	2	3

Abbreviations: FFR = fractional flow reserve; IVUS = intravascular ultrasound; OCT = optical coherence tomograph
*Prioritized topics (1–12) are listed in the order they were prioritized by the stakeholder panel.

High-Priority Future Research Needs Topic 1

What is the impact on clinical outcomes of a treatment decision (medical therapy, stent, or bypass) made on the basis of the adjunctive use of intravascular physiologic diagnostics, as compared with angiography alone?

Background

The CER evaluating intravascular diagnostic techniques identified evidence gaps pertaining to the use of these diagnostic techniques in diagnosing, assessing, and triaging patients with suspected CAD to appropriate therapeutic modalities (medical therapy, stent, or bypass). Only one trial rated as being low risk of bias compared the adjunctive use of intravascular physiologic diagnostics (FFR) versus angiography alone during stenting.[41] Although the evidence was rated to be of moderate strength, the stakeholders felt more research was needed for a number of reasons. First, as evidence currently rests primarily on one randomized controlled trial (RCT) there is the possibility that future studies will not support the favorable effect of FFR-guided stenting; this phenomenon, an initial effect that eventually dissipates through subsequent studies, has been well documented.[44] Second, given the widespread use of stents (with associated harms and costs) and the well documented variation in practice, any technology that can better target risks and benefits could have a major impact on patient outcomes and healthcare costs. As such it is important to fully explore dimensions beyond what is covered in existing trials. These include whether FFR should be applied to diagnose patients with suspected CAD and triage them to different therapeutic modalities (medical therapy, stent, or bypass) based on the results of intravascular physiologic diagnostics[e], how they apply to patients with borderline or intermediate lesions and other subgroups such as women (especially regarding the dilemma of non-obstructive CAD) and those with significant comorbidities, and how to use intravascular physiologic diagnostics to better characterize angiographic markers.[41,44]

Proposed Study Design

We propose a prospective observational study design, using a combination of catheterization registry data that are derived directly from electronic health records, linked with Medicare claims and state mortality records. Treatment assignment would be non-random, but statistical techniques could be used to adjust for potential confounding from treatment selection.

Value of Study Design

Even though an RCT comparing the use versus nonuse of FFR-guided angiography could help clarify the value of additional information from intravascular diagnostic to help determine which patients would benefit from optimal medical therapy, stent, or bypass graft, such an RCT may be difficult to conduct as FFR-guided PCI is fast-becoming the standard of care in patients with borderline and intermediate lesions (personal communication from M. Brennan).

While observational studies can compare outcomes of treatment decision made on the basis of FFR versus no FFR, they are subject to biases due to the lack of randomization. Established methodological approaches such as matching and regression analysis, including propensity score analyses, may be used to reduce biases from known imbalances at baseline. In addition,

---

[e]The recently published FAME II trial [NEJM 2012; 367:991-1001] suggests patients with stable CAD might benefit from the use of FFR. This trial did not have an angiography alone arm.

sensitivity analyses may be used to explore the robustness of findings for nonrandomized comparisons. However, the use of FFR depends on provider preference, which is subject to complex and difficult to measure factors. Thus, findings gleaned from cohort studies should be considered as hypothesis-generating rather than confirmatory.

On the other hand, observational studies have the benefit of wider generalizability when data collection occurs in real-life clinical settings and without restrictive inclusion criteria.

Ability To Recruit

There should be no barriers to recruitment for observational studies addressing the use of FFR.

Resource Use, Size, and Duration

The reliance on observational data substantially reduces resource use and increases feasibility in addressing this evidence gap. Post hoc analyses of existing observational studies can be done quickly and with modest resources. Generally, given the ease of retrospective data analysis, care should be taken to avoid biases from exploratory data-mining. Large databases like the National Cardiovascular Data Registry (NCDR) CathPCI Registry could be linked to Centers for Medicare and Medicaid (CMS) claims data;[45] this would provide data for comparative analyses of patients who had FFR versus those who had not.

Prospective observational studies allow for purposeful planning to answer hypotheses and more complete collection of relevant data, which can increase validity compared with post hoc observational studies using existing data. However, prospective planning and data collection consume a greater amount of resources.

Ethical Issues

There should be no ethical barriers to the analysis of existing databases or to conducting prospective trials in the investigation of this evidence gap. Patient confidentiality is assumed.

High-Priority Future Research Needs Topic 2

In patients with clinical or other indicators suggesting the potential need for revascularization (stenting or coronary bypass graft), even before the catheterization results are known, what is the impact on treatment decision (e.g., whether to stent); and stenting parameters (e.g., which lesion to stent, type of stent, stent length) of the use versus nonuse of intravascular diagnostics should the patients eventually undergo stenting? What is the impact on clinical outcomes?

2A. In patients with a high-risk positive stress perfusion scan (e.g., large areas of no or hypoperfusion in the myocardium), what is the impact on stenting parameters (e.g., which lesion to stent, type of stent, stent length) and clinical outcomes of the use versus nonuse of intravascular diagnostics if the patients undergo stenting?

2B. In patients with a negative stress perfusion scan but other precatheterization indicator like classic symptom complex suggesting the potential need for revascularization (stenting or coronary artery bypass graft), what is the impact on the decision to stent and clinical outcomes of the use versus non-use of intravascular diagnostics?

Background

The stakeholders raised the issue of the additional value of adjunctive intravascular diagnostic techniques in patients who already have either clinical or non-invasive diagnostic indication (e.g., high-risk positive stress perfusion scan) for undergoing stenting procedures or coronary artery bypass grafts. For those patients who are selected for stenting, one can hypothesize that additional information provided by intravascular diagnostics can aid in the selection of the type of stent, stent length, and other parameters in stent deployment. Our CER did not identify this as an evidence gap because our CER did not focus on this particular population. In addition, our CER evaluated the role of intravascular diagnostics only on the number of stents utilized and stent dilatation, but did not evaluate the role of intravascular diagnostics on the selection of the type of stent or stent length and how these choices impact clinical outcomes. This topic was further refined post survey into two subquestions 2A and 2B (see above) with the help of domain experts.

Proposed Study Designs

We propose both a prospective randomized controlled study and an observational study design. For this topic, our key informants informed us that FFR, a physiologic measurement, is primarily used in the determination of whether and which lesion to stent; while IVUS, an imaging technique, can aid in determining stent parameters like stent inflation pressure, stent length, and others. Accordingly, a pragmatic RCT can compare the use versus nonuse of IVUS in patients with a high-risk positive stress test, but an RCT comparing the use versus non-use of FFR-guided angiography may be difficult to conduct as FFR-guided PCI is fast-becoming the standard of care. We also propose a prospective observational study design, using a combination of catheterization registry data that are derived directly from electronic health records, linked with Medicare claims and state mortality records. Treatment assignment would be non-random, but statistical techniques could be used to adjust for potential confounding from treatment selection.

Randomized Controlled Trials

Value of Study Design

RCTs provide the most rigorous study design for examining comparative effectiveness for clinical outcomes. RCTs comparing the use of IVUS versus angiography alone on stenting parameters and clinical outcomes would help to fill in the evidence gaps. As it is unclear whether the real-world application will have similar results as RCT, trials should be pragmatic, with wide eligibility criteria and diverse settings. A reasonable time-frame for such studies would be 1 year or more. For a trial of IVUS versus no IVUS in patients with high-risk stress test results, it should be noted that medical therapy alone could still be a treatment option (in addition to stenting or coronary bypass) in both randomized arms, as our domain experts explained that for some of these patients, medical therapy alone may be appropriate.

Resource Use, Size, and Duration

An RCT, especially one with a long duration and large sample size, is a highly resource-intensive endeavor. The decision to conduct such a trial must be balanced against the value of the information that can be gained from longer followup and wider representation. It may be reasonable to design an RCT based on infrastructure already in place to minimize cost. For example, a pragmatic trial could be designed using the CathPCI registry.

To estimate an appropriate trial sample size, we carried out a power calculation using standard formula for a two-sided chi-square test. We based our effect size estimates on the actual estimates reported by Russo and colleagues' trial of IVUS versus angiography alone in patients scheduled for elective stent placements.[35] Assuming 1-year rates of target vessel revascularization (primary endpoint prespecified in the study) of 12 percent in the angiography group and 8 percent in the IVUS group, an alpha level of 0.05 and a statistical power of 0.80, a minimum sample size of 882 per group is required. As there was only a 7 percent attrition at 1 year for this trial, one could conservatively estimate loss to followup at no more than 5 to 10 percent with a diligent followup protocol. It should be noted that the Russo trial prespecified target vessel revascularization as the only primary endpoint. MACE is considered a secondary endpoint in this trial, estimates of which are similar and statistically nonsignificantly different between IVUS and angiography alone at 12 months (18.4 vs. 18.7 percent, respectively, P=0.93), suggesting powering our recommended trial based on patient outcomes from stenting may not be realistic.

Ability To Recruit

There could be barriers to recruitment for RCTs addressing this evidence gap as the use of intravascular diagnostics like IVUS gains wide acceptance.

Ethical Issues

As the use of the various intravascular diagnostic techniques becomes increasingly common in the community, there may not be a perceived equipoise to continue conducting trials of adjunctive intravascular diagnostics versus angiography alone despite the lack of studies demonstrating impact on patient outcomes.

Observational Studies

Value of Study Design

Observational studies could provide preliminary data comparing patients with negative stress test who had intravascular diagnostics versus those who had not. Depending on the results, there may be equipoise to justify an RCT in the future.

Ability to Recruit

There should be no barriers to recruitment for observational studies addressing the use of FFR and/or IVUS.

Resource Use, Size, and Duration

Once again, large databases like the National Cardiovascular Data Registry CathPCI Registry could be linked to Centers for Medicare and Medicaid (CMS) claims data;[45] this would provide data for comparative analyses of patients with negative stress test who had FFR or IVUS versus those who had not. Other databases like Mass-DAC (www.massdac.org) and New York State Percutaneous Coronary Intervention Reporting System (www.health.ny.gov/statistics/diseases/cardiovascular/docs/pci_2006-2008.pdf) could also provide useful comparative data.

Ethical issues

There should be no ethical barriers to the analysis of existing databases or to conducting prospective trials in the investigation of this evidence gap. Patient confidentiality is assumed.

High-Priority Future Research Needs Topic 3

Once the decision has been made to place a stent, what is the impact on clinical outcomes of the adjunctive use of intravascular imaging diagnostics, such as IVUS or optical coherence tomography (OCT), in stent placement and stent optimization, as compared with angiography alone?

Background

The CER evaluating intravascular imaging diagnostic techniques, such as IVUS or OCT, identified evidence gaps pertaining to the use of these diagnostic techniques in placement of newer stents and stent optimization, as compared with angiography. These newer stents can include drug-eluting stents, biodegradable stents, and others. Only two studies compared the adjunctive use of intravascular imaging diagnostics versus angiography alone during drug-eluting stent deployment.[18,19] There were no studies evaluating the adjunctive use of OCT versus angiography alone during stenting. Therefore, it is currently uncertain whether these techniques are effective in stent placement of newer stents and stent optimization, as compared with angiography.

Proposed Study Designs

We propose both a prospective randomized controlled study and an observational study design.

Randomized Controlled Trials

Value of Study Design

RCTs provide the most rigorous study design for examining comparative effectiveness for clinical outcomes. RCTs comparing the use of intravascular diagnostics versus angiography alone on stenting parameters and clinical outcomes would help to fill in the evidence gaps. As it is unclear whether the real-world application will have similar results as RCT, trials should be pragmatic, with wide eligibility criteria and diverse settings. A reasonable time-frame for such studies would be 1 year or more.

Resource Use, Size, and Duration

An RCT, especially one with a long duration and large sample size, is a highly resource-intensive endeavor. The decision to conduct such a trial must be balanced against the value of the information that can be gained from longer followup and wider representation. It may be reasonable to design an RCT based on infrastructure already in place to minimize cost. For example, a pragmatic trial could be designed using the CathPCI registry.

To estimate an appropriate trial sample size, we carried out a power calculation using standard formula for a two-sided chi-square test. We based our effect size estimates on the FAME trial.[41] Assuming 1-year rates of MACE of 18 percent in the angiography group and 13 percent in the FFR group, an alpha level of 0.05 and a statistical power of 0.80, a minimum sample size of 821 per group is required. As there was zero attrition at 1 year for the FAME trial, one could conservatively estimate loss to followup at no more than 5 to 10 percent with a diligent followup protocol.

Ability To Recruit

There could be barriers to recruitment for RCTs addressing this evidence gap as the use of intravascular diagnostics gains wide acceptance.

Ethical Issues

There may not be a perceived equipoise to continue conducting trials of adjunctive intravascular diagnostics versus angiography alone despite the lack of studies demonstrating impact on patient outcomes.

Observational Studies

Value of Study Design

Observational studies can compare outcomes of the use of intravascular diagnostics versus angiography alone. However, observational studies are subject to limitations described previously. However, the use of observational studies have the benefit of wider generalizability and likely to be a less costly proposition than an RCT.

Ability To Recruit

There should be no barriers to recruitment for observational studies addressing the use of intravascular diagnostics.

Resource Use, Size, and Duration

The reliance on observational data substantially reduces resource use and increases feasibility in addressing this evidence gap. However, existing registry like the CathPCI database does not have enough details to answer the questions concerning stenting parameters. A registry based on a collection of high volume centers specifically recording these details may have to be built de novo, thereby substantially increase the cost of this proposition. Alternatively, one could remunerate site investigators to pull and review cases to supplement details of interest to existing databases. For example, a novel module could be implemented in the CathPCI registry to collect additional IVUS parameters and additional stenting parameters. These data could be used to assess how IVUS influenced the procedure. This could be linked to the case file for the rest of the baseline and followup data and the non-IVUS PCI procedures from the registry could serve as the control.

Ethical Issues

There should be no ethical barriers to the analysis of existing databases or to conducting prospective trials in the investigation of this evidence gap. Patient confidentiality is assumed.

Discussion

Based on the 2012 intravascular diagnostic CER and our discussion with stakeholders, we identified 12 potential research areas, three of which were ranked as high priority areas of future research. Two topics (one on the use of intravascular physiologic measurements like fractional flow reserve in treatment decisionmaking before stenting; one on the impact of the use of intravascular imaging diagnostics on stenting) are based directly on evidence gaps identified in the CER. One topic on the added value of intravascular diagnostic techniques in patients with clear clinical and other indications for revascularization was raised by the stakeholders.

Our CER focused on the use of intravascular diagnostics and excluded noninvasive techniques. Therefore, evidence on the use of newer non-invasive techniques like chest computed tomography angiography with coronary computed tomography angiography (CCTA) in patients being considered for stenting has not been reviewed. The future research needs concerning the adjunctive use of noninvasive diagnostic techniques, perhaps in combination of invasive ones, will require a systematic evidence review and see what the gaps are.

The recommendations for priority topics for future research were generated based on a stakeholder-driven nomination and review process. We followed a recently developed taxonomy that was designed to aid researchers in the identification, recruitment and engagement of stakeholders. Our stakeholder panel represented a broad range of perspectives, across all major stakeholder categories identified in this taxonomy. Of 11 stakeholders who were invited, 10 participated in the teleconferences, and 9 participated in the prioritization process.

The use of intravascular diagnostics in patients being considered for percutaneous coronary artery stenting is a highly technical topic and requires considerable domain knowledge to appreciate how these adjunctive diagnostics aid traditional coronary artery catheterization and stenting. Added to this difficulty is the challenge of defining optimal stent placement; this concept has permeated the clinical community but standards have not been established.

To identify priority future research needs we sought and successfully incorporated insight from clinical experts as well as from insurance, hospital, patient and policy experts. Additionally, we have asked domain experts to review the description of the technical details concerning these diagnostic devices, to assure that it is faithful to the complex clinical details of intravascular diagnostic technology as applied to cardiovascular disease.

Conclusion

This report identifies three high-priority future research needs with regards to intravascular diagnostic techniques, as determined by a stakeholder panel. They are:

1. What is the impact on clinical outcomes of a treatment decision (medical therapy, stent, or bypass) made on the basis of the adjunctive use of intravascular physiologic diagnostics, as compared with angiography alone?

2. In patients in whom there is already a clear clinical and other noninvasive diagnostic indication suggesting the need for revascularization (stenting or coronary artery bypass graft), what is the impact on stenting parameters (e.g., which lesion to stent, type of stent, stent length) and clinical outcomes of the use versus non-use of intravascular diagnostics in those undergoing stenting?

3. Once the decision has been made to place a stent, what is the impact on clinical outcomes of the adjunctive use of intravascular imaging diagnostics, such as IVUS or OCT, in stent placement and stent optimization, as compared with angiography alone?

In summary, both data from pragmatic randomized controlled trials and properly adjusted observational studies could be used to fill in these gaps and help address these important clinical questions.

References

1. Concannon TW, Meissner P, Grunbaum JA, et al. A new taxonomy for stakeholder engagement in patient-centered outcomes research. J Gen Intern Med. 2012 Aug;27(8):985-91. PMID: 22528615.

2. Raman G. Intravascular Diagnostic Procedures and Imaging Techniques versus Angiography Alone: A Comparative Effectiveness Review. 2012. PMID: None.

3. Agostoni P, Valgimigli M, Van Mieghem CA, et al. Comparison of early outcome of percutaneous coronary intervention for unprotected left main coronary artery disease in the drug-eluting stent era with versus without intravascular ultrasonic guidance. American Journal of Cardiology. 2005 Mar 1;95(5):644-47. PMID: 15721110.

4. Ahmed K, Jeong MH, Chakraborty R, et al. Role of intravascular ultrasound in patients with acute myocardial infarction undergoing percutaneous coronary intervention. American Journal of Cardiology. 108(1):8-14, 2011 Jul 1. PMID: 21529735.

5. Albiero R, Rau T, Schluter M, et al. Comparison of immediate and intermediate-term results of intravascular ultrasound versus angiography-guided Palmaz-Schatz stent implantation in matched lesions. Circulation. 1997 Nov 4;96(9):2997-3005. PMID: 9386168.

6. Biondi-Zoccai G, Sheiban I, Romagnoli E, et al. Is intravascular ultrasound beneficial for percutaneous coronary intervention of bifurcation lesions? Evidence from a 4,314-patient registry. Clinical Research in Cardiology. 100(11):1021-8, 2011 Nov. PMID: 21701872.

7. Blasini R, Neumann FJ, Schmitt C, et al. Restenosis rate after intravascular ultrasound-guided coronary stent implantation. Catheterization & Cardiovascular Diagnosis. 1998 Aug;44(4):380-86. PMID: 9716200.

8. Choi JW, Goodreau LM, Davidson CJ. Resource utilization and clinical outcomes of coronary stenting: a comparison of intravascular ultrasound and angiographical guided stent implantation. American Heart Journal 2001 Jul;142(1):112-18. PMID: 11431666.

9. Claessen BE, Mehran R, Mintz GS, et al. Impact of intravascular ultrasound imaging on early and late clinical outcomes following percutaneous coronary intervention with drug-eluting stents.[Erratum appears in JACC Cardiovasc Interv. 2011 Nov;4(11):1255]. Jacc: Cardiovascular Interventions 4(9):974-81, 2011 Sep. PMID: 21939937.

10. Faulknier BA, Broce M, Baskerville S, et al. Clinical outcomes following IVUS-guided stent deployment in a community hospital. Journal of Invasive Cardiology. 2004 Jun;16(6):311-15. PMID: 15156000.

11. Fearon WF, Bornschein B, Tonino PA, et al. Economic evaluation of fractional flow reserve-guided percutaneous coronary intervention in patients with multivessel disease. Circulation. 2010 Dec 14;122(24):2545-50. PMID: 21126973.

12. Fitzgerald PJ, Oshima A, Hayase M, et al. Final results of the Can Routine Ultrasound Influence Stent Expansion (CRUISE) study. Circulation. 2000 Aug 1;102(5):523-30. PMID: 10920064.

13. Frey AW, Hodgson JM, Muller C, et al. Ultrasound-guided strategy for provisional stenting with focal balloon combination catheter: results from the randomized Strategy for Intracoronary Ultrasound-guided PTCA and Stenting (SIPS) trial. Circulation. 2000 Nov 14;102(20):2497-502. PMID: 11076823.

14. Fujimoto H, Tao S, Dohi T, et al. Primary and mid-term outcome of sirolimus-eluting stent implantation with angiographic guidance alone. Journal of Cardiology. 2008 Feb;51(1):18-24. PMID: 18522771.

15. Gaster AL, Slothuus U, Larsen J, et al. Cost-effectiveness analysis of intravascular ultrasound guided percutaneous coronary intervention versus conventional percutaneous coronary intervention. Scandinavian Cardiovascular Journal. 2001 Mar;35(2):80-85. PMID: 11405501.

16. Gaster AL, Slothuus SU, Larsen J, et al. Continued improvement of clinical outcome and cost effectiveness following intravascular ultrasound guided PCI: insights from a prospective, randomised study. Heart. 2003 Sep;89(9):1043-49. PMID: 12923023.

17. Gerber RT, Latib A, Ielasi A, et al. Defining a new standard for IVUS optimized drug eluting stent implantation: the PRAVIO study. Catheterization & Cardiovascular Interventions. 2009 Aug 1;74(2):348-56. PMID: 19213067.

18. Gil RJ, Pawlowski T, Dudek D, et al. Comparison of angiographically guided direct stenting technique with direct stenting and optimal balloon angioplasty guided with intravascular ultrasound. The multicenter, randomized trial results. American Heart Journal. 2007 Oct;154(4):669-75. PMID: 17892989.

19. Jakabcin J, Spacek R, Bystron M, et al. Long-term health outcome and mortality evaluation after invasive coronary treatment using drug eluting stents with or without the IVUS guidance. Randomized control trial. HOME DES IVUS. Catheterization & Cardiovascular Interventions. 2010 Mar 1;75(4):578-83. PMID: 19902491.

20. Kawata M, Okada T, Igarashi N, et al. Assessment of intravascular ultrasound-bearing balloon catheter-guided percutaneous transluminal coronary angioplasty and stenting. Heart & Vessels. 1997;Suppl:12-17. PMID: 9476578.

21. Kim JS, Hong MK, Ko YG, et al. Impact of intravascular ultrasound guidance on long-term clinical outcomes in patients treated with drug-eluting stent for bifurcation lesions: data from a Korean multicenter bifurcation registry. American Heart Journal. 2011 Jan;161(1):180-87. PMID: 21167352.

22. Maluenda G, Lemesle G, Ben-Dor I, et al. Impact of intravascular ultrasound guidance in patients with acute myocardial infarction undergoing percutaneous coronary intervention. Catheterization & Cardiovascular Interventions. 2010 Jan 1;75(1):86-92. PMID: 19670305.

23. Mudra H, Di MC, de JP, et al. Randomized comparison of coronary stent implantation under ultrasound or angiographic guidance to reduce stent restenosis (OPTICUS Study). Circulation. 2001 Sep 18;104(12):1343-49. PMID: 11560848.

24. Mueller C, Mc Hodgson JB, Brutsche M, et al. Impact of intracoronary ultrasound guidance on long-term outcome of percutaneous coronary interventions in diabetics--insights from the randomized SIPS trial. Swiss Medical Weekly. 2002 Jun 1;132(21-22):279-84. PMID: 12362285.

25. Muramatsu T, Tsukahara R, Ho M, et al. Usefulness of fractional flow reserve guidance for PCI in acute myocardial infarction. Journal of Invasive Cardiology. 2002 Nov;14(11):657-62. PMID: 12403892.

26. Nam CW, Yoon HJ, Cho YK, et al. Outcomes of percutaneous coronary intervention in intermediate coronary artery disease: fractional flow reserve-guided versus intravascular ultrasound-guided. Jacc: Cardiovascular Interventions. 2010 Aug; 3(8):812-17. PMID: 20723852.

27. Nasu K, Tsuchikane E, Awata N, et al. Quantitative angiographic and intravascular ultrasound study >5 years after directional coronary atherectomy. American Journal of Cardiology. 2004 Mar 1;93(5):543-48. PMID: 14996576.

28. Oemrawsingh PV, Mintz GS, Schalij MJ, et al. Intravascular ultrasound guidance improves angiographic and clinical outcome of stent implantation for long coronary artery stenoses: final results of a randomized comparison with angiographic guidance (TULIP Study). Circulation. 2003 Jan 7;107(1):62-67. PMID: 12515744.

29. Orford JL, Denktas AE, Williams BA, et al. Routine intravascular ultrasound scanning guidance of coronary stenting is not associated with improved clinical outcomes. American Heart Journal. 2004 Sep;148(3):501-06. PMID: 15389239.

30. Ozaki Y, Yamaguchi T, Suzuki T, et al. Impact of cutting balloon angioplasty (CBA) prior to bare metal stenting on restenosis. Circulation Journal. 2007 Jan;71(1):1-8. PMID: 17186970.

31. Park SJ, Hong MK, Lee CW, et al. Elective stenting of unprotected left main coronary artery stenosis: effect of debulking before stenting and intravascular ultrasound guidance. Journal of the American College of Cardiology. 2001 Oct;38(4):1054-60. PMID: 11583882.

32. Park SJ, Kim YH, Park DW, et al. Impact of intravascular ultrasound guidance on long-term mortality in stenting for unprotected left main coronary artery stenosis. Circulation: Cardiovascular Interventions. 2009 Jun;2(3):167-77. PMID: 20031713.

33. Pijls NH, Fearon WF, Tonino PA, et al. Fractional flow reserve versus angiography for guiding percutaneous coronary intervention in patients with multivessel coronary artery disease: 2-year follow-up of the FAME (Fractional Flow Reserve Versus Angiography for Multivessel Evaluation) study. Journal of the American College of Cardiology. 2010 Jul 13;56(3):177-84. PMID: 20537493.

34. Roy P, Steinberg DH, Sushinsky SJ, et al. The potential clinical utility of intravascular ultrasound guidance in patients undergoing percutaneous coronary intervention with drug-eluting stents. European Heart Journal. 2008 Aug;29(15):1851-57. PMID: 18550555.

35. Russo RJ, Silva PD, Teirstein PS, et al. A randomized controlled trial of angiography versus intravascular ultrasound-directed bare-metal coronary stent placement (the AVID Trial). Circulation: Cardiovascular Interventions. 2009 Apr;2(2):113-23. PMID: 20031704.

36. Sakamoto T, Kawarabayashi T, Taguchi H, et al. Intravascular ultrasound-guided balloon angioplasty for treatment of in-stent restenosis. Catheterization & Cardiovascular Interventions. 1999 Jul;47(3):298-303. PMID: 10402282.

37. Schiele F, Meneveau N, Vuillemenot A, et al. Impact of intravascular ultrasound guidance in stent deployment on 6-month restenosis rate: a multicenter, randomized study comparing two strategies--with and without intravascular ultrasound guidance. RESIST Study Group. REStenosis after Ivus guided STenting. Journal of the American College of Cardiology. 1998 Aug;32(2):320-28. PMID: 9708456.

38. Schiele F, Meneveau N, Seronde MF, et al. Medical costs of intravascular ultrasound optimization of stent deployment. Results of the multicenter randomized 'REStenosis after Intravascular ultrasound STenting' (RESIST) study. Int J Cardiovasc Intervent. 2000 Dec;3(4):207-13. PMID: 12431345.

39. Seo T, Yamao K, Hayashi T, et al. [Intravascular ultrasound in determining the end point of percutaneous transluminal coronary angioplasty]. [Japanese]. Journal of Cardiology. 1996 Oct;28(4):183-89. PMID: 8934333.

40. Talley JD, Mauldin PD, Becker ER, et al. Cost and therapeutic modification of intracoronary ultrasound-assisted coronary angioplasty. American Journal of Cardiology. 1996 Jun 15;77(15):1278-82. PMID: 8677866.

41. Tonino PA, De BB, Pijls NH, et al. Fractional flow reserve versus angiography for guiding percutaneous coronary intervention. New England Journal of Medicine. 2009 Jan 15;360(3):213-24. PMID: 19144937.

42. Wongpraparut N, Yalamanchili V, Pasnoori V, et al. Thirty-month outcome after fractional flow reserve-guided versus conventional multivessel percutaneous coronary intervention. American Journal of Cardiology. 2005 Oct 1;96(7):877-84. PMID: 16188509.

43. Yoshitomi Y, Kojima S, Yano M, et al. Benefit of intravascular ultrasound in Wiktor stent implantation. Catheterization & Cardiovascular Interventions. 1999 May;47(1):28-35. PMID: 10385154.

44. Ioannidis JP, Ntzani EE, Trikalinos TA, et al. Replication validity of genetic association studies. Nat Genet. 2001 Nov;29(3):306-09. PMID: 11600885.

45.   Brennan JM, Peterson ED, Messenger JC, et al. Linking the National Cardiovascular Data Registry CathPCI Registry with Medicare claims data: validation of a longitudinal cohort of elderly patients undergoing cardiac catheterization. Circ Cardiovasc Qual Outcomes. 2012 Jan;5(1):134-40. PMID: 22253370.

Acronyms

AHRQ	Agency for Healthcare Research and Quality
CABG	Coronary artery bypass graft surgery
CAD	Coronary artery disease
CER	Comparative Effectiveness Review
CMS	Centers for Medicare and Medicaid Services
EHC	Effective Health Care
EPC	Evidence-based Practice Center
EMS	Emergency Medical Services
FDA	Food and Drug Administration (U.S.)
FFR	Fractional flow reserve
FRN	Future Research Needs
IVUS	Intravascular ultrasound
KQ	Key Question
LMD	Left main (coronary artery) disease
MACE	Major adverse cardiac event
MI	Myocardial infarction
NCDR	National Cardiovascular Data Registry
OCT	Optical coherence tomography
PCI	Percutaneous coronary intervention
PICOD	Population, Intervention, Comparator, Outcome, study Design
QCA	Quantitative coronary angiography
RCT	Randomized controlled trial
STEMI	ST-segment elevation myocardial infarction
TEP	Technical Expert Panel
TLR	Target lesion revascularization
TOO	Task Order Officer

Appendix A. Effective Health Care Program Selection Criteria

Appropriateness:
- Represents a health care drug, intervention, device, technology or health care system/setting available (or soon to be available) in the United States.
- Relevant to 1013 enrollees (Medicare, Medicaid, S-CHIP, other Federal health care programs.
- Represents one of the priority conditions designated by the U.S. Department of Health and Human Services (HHS).

Importance:
- Represents a significant disease burden, large proportion or priority population.
- Is of high public interest; affects health care decision-making, outcomes, or costs for a large proportion of the U.S. population or for a priority population in particular.
- Was nominated/strongly supported by one or more stakeholder groups.
- Represents important uncertainty for decisionmakers.
- Incorporates issues around both clinical benefits and potential clinical harms.
- Represents important variation in clinical care, or controversy in what constitutes appropriate clinical care.
- Represent high costs to consumers, patients, health care systems or payers; due to common use, high unit costs, or high associated costs.

Desirability of New Research/Duplication:
- Would not be redundant (i.e., the proposed topic is not already covered by available or soon-to-be available evidence.)

Feasibility:
- Effectively uses existing research and knowledge by considering adequacy of research for conducting research, and newly available evidence.

Potential Impact:
- Potential for significant health impact, significant economic impact, potential change, potential risk from inaction, addressing inequities and vulnerable populations, and/or addressing a topic with clear implications for resolving important dilemmas in health and health care decisions made by one or more stakeholder groups.